KNOWLEDGE GUIDE TO OSTEOPOROSIS

Essential Manual To Prevention, Diagnosis, And Treatment Strategies For Stronger And Improved Bone Health

DR. AARON BRANUM

Copyright © 2024 BY DR. AARON BRANUM

All rights reserved. Except for brief quotations embodied in critical reviews and certain other noncommercial uses permitted by copyright law, no part of this publication may be reproduced, distributed, or transmitted in any form or by any means, Including photocopying, recording, or other electronic or mechanical methods, without the prior written permission of the publisher.

Disclaimer:

The data in this book, is solely meant to be informative and instructional.

This book is not intended to replace expert medical advice, diagnosis, or care. No medical, health, or other professional services are offered by the author, publisher, or any affiliated parties

Individual outcomes may differ in the practice of these therapies, which entail a variety of approaches and methodologies.

A one-on-one session with a trained or certified healthcare professional is still preferable. It is best to consult a trained healthcare provider before making any decisions regarding your health.

The author of this book is not affiliated with any specific website, product, or organization related to any of these therapies.

All reasonable measures have been taken by the author and publisher to guarantee the authenticity and dependability of the material contained in this book

Contents

CHAPTER ONE 13
  SMALL BASICS 13
    Bone Anatomy 13
    Strength And Density Of Bones 14
    Affecting Factors For Bone Health 15
    The Value Of Vitamin D And Calcium 16
    Developing Healthy Bones At Any Age 17

CHAPTER TWO 21
  OSTEOPOROSIS DIAGNOSIS 21
    Tests For Bone Density: What To Expect .. 21
    Analysing Bone Density Data 22
    Comprehending Z- And T-Scores 24
    Other Examinations To Determine Bone Health 25
    When To Consult A Physician 26

CHAPTER THREE 29
  RISK ELEMENTS AND ACTIONS 29
    Finding Osteoporosis Risk Factors 29
    Lifestyle Modifications For Healthy Bones . 30

Exercise's Key Role In Osteoporosis
　　Prevention 31
　　Dietary Advice For Strong Bones 32
　　Steer Clear Of Bone-Damaging Habits......33
CHAPTER FOUR 35
　OPTIONS FOR TREATMENT 35
　　Treatments For Osteoporosis Drugs.........35
　　Hormone Therapy: Benefits And Drawbacks
　　..36
　　Changing One's Lifestyle As A Treatment..37
　　Surgical Procedures For Serious Instances 38
　　Alternative And Complementary Medicine.39
CHAPTER FIVE 41
　OSTEOPOROSIS: A LIVING CONDITION 41
　　Managing Physical Restrictions................41
　　Advice On Preventing Falls 43
　　Changing Your Home To Increase Safety..46
　　Keeping Yourself Independent Despite
　　Osteoporosis 49
　　Asking For Help From Family And Friends
　　And Medical Experts 51

CHAPTER SIX 55
OSTEOPOROSIS AND EXERCISE 55
Exercises That Are Good for Bone Health .. 55
Establishing A Secure Workout Schedule .. 57
Exercise Guidelines For People With Osteoporosis 59
Combining Strength And Balance Training 61

CHAPTER SEVEN 67
SUMMARY AND EXPOSURE TO CANCER 67
Foods And Supplements High In Calcium .. 67
Sources And Dosages Of Vitamin D 68
Protein's Importance For Healthy Bones ... 69
Foods To Restrict Or Stay Away From 70
Organising Meals For Maximum Bone Strength 71

CHAPTER EIGHT 73
OVERCOMING OSTEOPOROSIS AT DIFFERENT PHASES OF LIFE 73
Osteoporosis In Adolescents And Children 73
Young Adults And Middle-Aged People's Osteoporosis 76

Osteoporosis During Breastfeeding And Pregnancy 80

Osteoporosis In Seniors And Older Adults . 84

CHAPTER NINE 89

COMMON QUESTIONS AND ANSWERS 89

Is It Possible To Regain Bone Mass? 89

Do Any All-Natural Treatments For Osteoporosis? 90

How Do Guys Get Osteoporosis? 91

Can Osteoporosis Be Inherited? 92

What Recent Developments Exist In The Field Of Osteoporosis Research? 94

ABOUT THIS BOOK

The importance of "Knowledge Guide to Osteoporosis" goes well beyond a book; it is a source of knowledge in a field that is frequently cloaked in misunderstandings and confusion. Fundamentally, it is a thorough investigation of osteoporosis, revealing its secrets and illuminating its complex network of ramifications.

The book deftly explains the fundamentals of bone health, demystifying terms like bone density, strength, and the vital roles of calcium and vitamin D. It starts with an introductory tour of the architecture of bones. An exploration of the variables that affect bone health, enables readers to understand the complex relationship between lifestyle decisions and skeletal integrity, encouraging a proactive strategy for maintaining bone density throughout life.

The book proves to be a reliable guide as it helps readers navigate the maze of diagnostics, clarifying the subtleties of bone density tests and deciphering the mysterious language of T- and Z-scores. It gives readers the knowledge they need to interpret test findings and make wise decisions regarding their bone health with clarity and precision.

As the story progresses, the book addresses risk factors and prevention techniques head-on, providing a road map for strengthening skeletal resilience through nutritional interventions, exercise routines, and lifestyle changes. It acts as a protector, keeping watch on the growing flood of behaviors that erode bone structure and welcoming the diverse array of available treatments, which include prescription drugs, surgery, and complementary therapies.

However, "Knowledge Guide to Osteoporosis" goes beyond academic discussion and offers guidance for day-to-day living. It turns into a ray of hope for people suffering from the psychological and physical effects of osteoporosis, providing helpful guidance on coping strategies, preventing falls, and cultivating independence in the face of hardship.

Furthermore, the book promotes empowerment rather than just knowledge. It becomes a catalyst for change by examining workout regimens designed to support bone health and dietary tactics meant to strengthen skeletal integrity, encouraging readers to take back control of their own health.

The book offers a continuity thread through the stages of life, covering the particular issues and concerns associated with osteoporosis in different generations. From youth to old age, it is a constant friend, providing wise counsel and customized insights.

Ultimately, "Knowledge Guide to Osteoporosis" is proof of the ability of information to drive out fear and promote resilience.

It serves as a beacon of hope, empowerment, and understanding for individuals navigating the maze of osteoporosis by illuminating frequently asked questions and providing answers.

CHAPTER ONE

SMALL BASICS

Bone Anatomy

Our bodies' strong skeleton, made up of bones, gives our important organs shape, support, and protection. To understand how they work and stay healthy, one must be aware of their anatomy. The living tissues that give bones their strength and flexibility are collagen and calcium phosphate. They are dynamic, not static, structures that are always changing and adjusting to different stresses.

Bone marrow is the place where blood cells are made, and a system of blood arteries that carry oxygen and nutrients are found inside bones. The layers that make up a bone are formed of compact bone on the outside and spongy bone, which is lighter and has a porous structure, inside. Because of its complex structure, which strikes a balance between strength and lightness, bones can tolerate strain and absorb shocks.

Strength And Density Of Bones

The quantity of minerals present in bone tissue is referred to as bone density. It's a vital sign of bone health since stronger, less likely to-break bones are denser bones.

The late 20s are usually when bone density reaches its peak, after which it progressively decreases. Osteoporosis, a disorder marked by porous and brittle bones, can result from lifestyle choices and medical disorders that hasten this decline.

A fine balance between bone creation and resorption—the breakdown and replacement of old bone tissue with new—is necessary to maintain ideal bone density. Weight-bearing activities, like strength training or walking, promote the growth of new bones, and bone mineralization is supported by a diet high in calcium and vitamin D. Maintaining bone density and strength over the course of a lifetime requires both regular exercise and a diet rich in key nutrients.

Affecting Factors For Bone Health

Bone health is influenced by a number of variables, including lifestyle choices and genetics. Bone form and density are largely determined by genetics, but other lifestyle factors including nutrition, exercise, and sun exposure also have a big impact. Hormonal fluctuations can impact bone density and remodeling, especially during puberty and menopause.

Bone health may be compromised by specific medical disorders and drugs. For example, bone loss can be accelerated by diseases like rheumatoid arthritis or hormone imbalances, and over time, drugs like corticosteroids can weaken bones. Furthermore, smoking and binge drinking have a negative impact on bone density, raising the possibility of osteoporosis and fractures.

The Value Of Vitamin D And Calcium

The nutrients calcium and vitamin D are crucial for healthy bones. The main mineral that gives bones their strength and structure is calcium, which is facilitated in its absorption and use by vitamin D.

Insufficient amounts of these nutrients can cause bones to weaken and fracture more easily, raising the risk of osteoporosis and fractures.

Calcium may be found in abundance in dairy products, almonds, leafy greens, and fortified meals.

On the other hand, vitamin D can be acquired from sunlight exposure and certain foods, such as fatty fish and fortified foods. However a lot of people might not obtain enough of these nutrients from their food alone, so supplements are usually necessary, especially for those who are susceptible to deficiencies.

Developing Healthy Bones At Any Age

The process of developing and keeping strong bones starts in childhood and lasts into maturity.

A healthy diet and regular exercise are essential for developing appropriate bone mass during the crucial stages of childhood and adolescence.

The foundation for lifetime bone health is laid by encouraging kids to participate in regular physical exercise and eat a balanced diet high in calcium and vitamin D.

But investing in bone health is something you can do at any time. Adopting good living choices can help preserve bone density and lower the risk of osteoporosis even as one ages into adulthood and beyond.

Walking, running, and dancing are examples of weight-bearing workouts that promote the creation of new bones, whereas resistance training fortifies existing muscles and bones.

Furthermore, maintaining sufficient calcium and vitamin D intake through food or supplements promotes the health of our bones as we age.

Through proactive steps and a focus on bone health, people can reduce their risk of osteoporosis and preserve strong, robust bones for the duration of their lives.

CHAPTER TWO

OSTEOPOROSIS DIAGNOSIS

Tests For Bone Density: What To Expect

The strength and density of your bones can be determined with non-invasive bone density examinations. Dual-energy X-ray absorptiometry (DXA) scans are usually used in these exams, and they are quick and painless.

You will lie on a table during the exam, and a machine will scan particular parts of your body, mainly your hips, forearms, and spine. There is very little radiation utilized, and it is deemed safe.

You may be required to wear loose-fitting clothing, take out any metal objects that could interfere with the scan, and stop taking calcium supplements for a specific amount of time before the test. When you're prepared, the technician will carefully position you and start the scan. For the operation to be accurate, you must remain motionless.

You can get right back to your regular activities after the exam. Your doctor can evaluate the state of your bones and talk about any necessary treatment or lifestyle modifications once the results are usually available soon after the scan.

Analysing Bone Density Data

It is essential to comprehend your bone density results in order to evaluate your osteoporosis risk and choose the best course of action.

T- and Z-scores are commonly used to express the findings of a bone density test.

T-scores measure how much bone density you have in comparison to a healthy, gender-neutral young adult.

Low bone mass (osteopenia) is indicated by a T-score between -1 and -2.5, while a T-score between +1 and -1 is regarded as normal. When a T-score is -2.5 or below, osteoporosis is present.

Conversely, Z-scores allow you to compare your bone density to others who are similar to you in terms of size, gender, and age.

These ratings may be used to determine underlying diseases or other elements influencing bone health.

To establish the best course of therapy, your doctor will evaluate the findings of your bone density test in combination with information from your medical history, lifestyle, and family history of osteoporosis.

Comprehending Z- And T-Scores

Osteoporosis diagnosis and bone health assessment are greatly aided by T- and Z-scores. Z-scores compare your bone density to people your own age, gender, and size, whereas T-scores compare it to that of a healthy young adult.

You can assume that your bone density is within the usual range for a young, healthy adult if your T-score falls between +1 and -1. Low bone mass, or osteopenia, is indicated by a T-score of -1 to -2.5, which increases the chance of developing osteoporosis.

If your T-score is -2.5 or below, you have osteoporosis, which means your bones are more weaker and more likely to break.

Z-scores, however, contrast your bone density with that of people in your age range.

If your Z-score is less than -2.0, it can mean that you have less bone density than you should for your age and that there may be underlying issues affecting the health of your bones.

Other Examinations To Determine Bone Health

Other tests may be performed in addition to bone density examinations to evaluate bone health and pinpoint possible osteoporosis risk factors.

These tests include hormone testing to evaluate thyroid function and hormone levels, as well as blood tests to monitor calcium and vitamin D levels.

A variety of imaging procedures, including MRIs, CT scans, and X-rays, can be used to assess bone structure and spot any anomalies or fractures.

These examinations can give important details about the condition of your bones and assist your physician in creating a personalized treatment strategy.

When To Consult A Physician

It's critical to visit a physician for an assessment and necessary tests if you have risk factors for osteoporosis, such as a family history of the condition, or if you are exhibiting symptoms.

Osteoporosis symptoms might include low bone mass, low bone density, and low-force fractures.

It's also advised to talk to your doctor about bone health if you're older than 50, particularly if you have risk factors like smoking, binge drinking, or leading a sedentary lifestyle.

In order to manage osteoporosis and lower the risk of consequences like fractures, early detection and management are essential.

CHAPTER THREE
RISK ELEMENTS AND ACTIONS
Finding Osteoporosis Risk Factors

There are not always warning signs for osteoporosis. It can be crucial to recognize the risk factors in order to stop it from starting.

Age plays a big role; as we age, our bone density gradually declines, increasing the risk of fractures.

Reduced estrogen puts women at greater risk, particularly those who have gone through menopause. Genetics also play a part; you may be prone to osteoporosis if your family has a history of the condition.

A sedentary lifestyle, smoking, and heavy alcohol use are examples of lifestyle variables that might hasten the loss of bone mass. The risk can also be raised by some drugs, such as corticosteroids, and medical disorders, such as rheumatoid arthritis.

Lifestyle Modifications For Healthy Bones

Making small lifestyle changes can have a significant impact on maintaining bone health. It's critical to stop smoking since it affects the body's ability to absorb calcium and weakens bones.

Alcohol use should be controlled as well, as too much of it can disrupt bone growth and raise the risk of fractures. Bone strength is enhanced by weight-bearing workouts including jogging, dancing, and walking.

Increased bone density can also be achieved through resistance training using weights or resistance bands. It's important to maintain a healthy weight because obesity can put stress on the bones and joints and being underweight can raise the chance of fractures.

Exercise's Key Role In Osteoporosis Prevention

Exercise is essential for maintaining strong, healthy bones in addition to helping you stay in shape. Exercises involving weight bearing, which forces muscles and bones to defy gravity, are especially good for bone health. These include activities like walking, hiking, jogging, and stair climbing.

By encouraging the growth of new bone tissue, these activities improve bone strength and density. Resistance workouts, such as lifting weights or utilizing resistance bands, help in growing muscle mass, which indirectly improves bone health.

Even hobbies like yoga and tai chi, which enhance balance and coordination, can lessen the chance of falls and fractures, therefore protecting bone health.

Dietary Advice For Strong Bones

A balanced diet plays a significant part in maintaining optimal bone health. Calcium is a cornerstone; add calcium-rich foods like dairy products, leafy greens, almonds, and fortified foods to your diet.

Because it facilitates the body's absorption of calcium, vitamin D is similarly vital. To ensure you receive enough of it, get outside and eat foods high in vitamin D, such as egg yolks, fatty fish, and fortified cereals.

Lean meats, chicken, fish, beans, and lentils are good sources of protein, which is necessary for the development and maintenance of bones. For strong bones, you also need to consume a diet high in fruits, vegetables, whole grains, nuts, and seeds, as well as magnesium, phosphorus, vitamin K, and vitamin C.

Steer Clear Of Bone-Damaging Habits

Avoiding certain habits is essential to preventing osteoporosis since they can negatively impact your bone health.

The number one habit is smoking, which not only weakens bones but also obstructs the absorption of calcium and other vital nutrients. Overindulgence in alcohol is another factor that contributes to bone loss; keep your consumption to reasonable amounts.

Limit your intake of coffee and tea since excessive caffeine use can also cause calcium to be lost from bones. Make balanced, nutrient-dense meals your preference instead of crash or extreme diets, which can deprive your body of vital nutrients needed for healthy bones.

Finally, to maintain strong and healthy bones, try to avoid sitting for extended periods of time and instead stand up, stretch, and move around frequently.

CHAPTER FOUR

OPTIONS FOR TREATMENT

For effective treatment, osteoporosis—a disorder marked by weakening bones—needs to be approached from several angles. Options for treatment include a variety of approaches, such as medication, lifestyle changes, and, in extreme circumstances, surgery.

Treatments For Osteoporosis Drugs

Osteoporosis medications are essential because they slow down bone loss and lower the chance of fracture. Bisphosphonates are one type of medication that is frequently used for this use. By preventing bone deterioration, these drugs contribute to the preservation of bone density. Risedronate, ibandronate, and alendronate are a few examples. Selective estrogen receptor modulators (SERMs) are a different class of drug that works by imitating the effects of estrogen in the body, which helps to stop bone loss. One SERM that is frequently given for the treatment of osteoporosis is raloxifene.

In order to preserve bone density, hormone replacement therapy (HRT) may also be suggested for postmenopausal women. However, there are possible dangers and advantages associated with HRT use, which should be carefully evaluated in collaboration with a healthcare professional.

Hormone Therapy: Benefits And Drawbacks

Osteoporosis has long been managed with hormone therapy, specifically estrogen replacement therapy, especially in postmenopausal women. The reduction of estrogen during menopause can exacerbate bone loss because it is essential for preserving bone density. Hormone therapy can lessen the chance of osteoporotic fractures and help with menopausal symptoms.

However, since hormone therapy has been linked to a higher risk of some medical conditions, including blood clots and breast cancer, it's crucial to balance the possible advantages against the risks. Hormone therapy is therefore usually only advised for brief periods of time and may not be appropriate for every person.

Changing One's Lifestyle As A Treatment

Treatment for osteoporosis must include lifestyle changes in addition to medicines. Frequent weight-bearing exercises, including jogging, walking, or resistance training, help build stronger bones and enhance balance, which lowers the chance of fractures and falls. It's also essential to consume enough calcium and vitamin D to keep your bones healthy. Dairy products, leafy greens, and fortified foods are high in calcium. Supplementing with vitamin D and getting enough sunshine will also help. It's critical to abstain from smoking and heavy alcohol use since these behaviors can erode bone density and raise the risk of fracture.

Surgical Procedures For Serious Instances

To regain mobility and stop further difficulties, surgical procedures may be required for people with severe osteoporosis or those who have suffered crippling fractures.

Vertebroplasty and kyphoplasty, which entail injecting bone cement into fractured vertebrae to stabilize them and ease pain, are common surgical procedures for osteoporosis. Joint replacement surgery may be necessary in certain situations to replace damaged joints, like the hip or knee, with artificial implants.

These surgical procedures are usually saved for patients whose osteoporosis-related fractures significantly limit their ability to carry out everyday activities and who have not reacted well to conservative therapy.

Alternative And Complementary Medicine

Complementary and alternative therapies may be beneficial for controlling osteoporosis in addition to traditional medical therapy. These treatments frequently emphasize holistic methods to support general health and well-being. For instance, research has examined how acupuncture, massage therapy, and yoga may help people with osteoporosis feel less stressed, move more freely, and manage their pain.

Before adding any complementary or alternative therapies to your osteoporosis treatment plan, you should speak with a healthcare professional because their safety and efficacy can vary and they should be used in addition to conventional medical care rather than as a replacement.

CHAPTER FIVE

OSTEOPOROSIS: A LIVING CONDITION

Managing Physical Restrictions

Managing physical limits is a common aspect of living with osteoporosis. Individual differences in the severity of the illness and other circumstances may cause these limits to differ from person to person. However typical problems include discomfort, decreased mobility, and a higher risk of fractures. Nevertheless, coping mechanisms can greatly enhance life satisfaction.

First and foremost, adopting an attitude of acceptance and flexibility is crucial. Finding new methods to complete chores and participate in activities is what it means to accept physical limitations instead of giving up. This could involve changing daily habits to lessen stress on weakening bones or utilizing assistive devices like walkers or canes to help with movement.

Exercise is essential for managing the physical restrictions brought on by osteoporosis. Although high-impact exercises may be avoided because of the possibility of fractures, low-impact activities like swimming, tai chi, or walking can help maintain bone density, enhance balance, and build muscle. Exercises that are safe and customized to each person's needs can be ensured by working with a physical therapist or professional trainer.

Additionally, using proper body mechanics and posture helps lessen the load on weaker bones and joints. Easy fixes like straightening your posture, lifting objects correctly, and avoiding abrupt twisting motions can reduce pain and prevent injuries.

Taking care of the psychological and emotional parts of coping is just as vital as the physical strategies.

Mental health can suffer when one is dealing with physical limits or chronic pain. In order to manage stress and foster emotional resilience, one can consider seeking therapy, joining support groups, or practicing relaxation techniques like deep breathing exercises or meditation.

Advice On Preventing Falls

For those who have osteoporosis, preventing falls is crucial since fractures from falls can have dangerous repercussions. Thankfully, there are a number of tactics that help lower the chance of fractures and lower the danger of falls.

Making your home a safe place is one of the best ways to prevent falls. This includes clearing away clutter and loose carpets to prevent trips and falls, adding grab bars to stairwells and restrooms, and making sure the entire house has enough illumination. Non-slip mats in the shower and bathtub can also help to prevent mishaps.

An additional important component of fall prevention is maintaining strength and balance through regular exercise. Exercises aimed at enhancing muscular strength, flexibility, and balance can assist people respond to loss of balance and avoid falls.

Yoga poses and other balancing exercises, such as standing on one leg, might be especially helpful.

Since some medications might make you drowsy or dizzy, which increases your risk of falling, medication management is also crucial for preventing falls. It's crucial to routinely go over prescriptions with a medical expert and go over any possible interactions or negative effects.

Putting on supportive, well-fitting shoes with non-slip soles is another easy yet powerful fall-prevention strategy. Sturdy soles and low heels give stability and lessen the chance of slipping.

And last, falling can be avoided by being aware of your surroundings and always watchful. Accident risk can be considerably decreased by being aware of potential hazards and adopting preventative measures, such as using handrails when climbing or descending stairs.

Changing Your Home To Increase Safety

It is imperative that homes be adapted to improve accessibility and safety for those who have osteoporosis. Easy adjustments can have a big influence on minimizing the effects of physical limitations and falling risk.

For people with osteoporosis, installing grab bars and handrails in strategic locations like restrooms, stairwells, and hallways can offer stability and support.

These fixtures make it possible to move more safely and lower the risk of accidents, especially in places where there are tripping or slipping hazards.

Furthermore, a clear and secure environment can be created by clearing debris and obstructions out of living areas and passageways.

This includes fastening unsecured carpets, arranging furniture to facilitate simple movement, and keeping frequently used things close at hand to reduce the need for bending or stretching.

Increasing the lighting in the entire house is another essential safety change. Having enough lighting lowers the chance of trips and falls, particularly at night or in poorly lit locations.

Adding motion-sensor lighting to outside walkways and halls can improve security and visibility as well.

Apart from alterations to their structure, the integration of assistive gadgets and adaptive equipment can enhance the autonomy and security of people suffering from osteoporosis.

This could include adding an elevated toilet seat for easy access, taking baths in a shower chair or bench, or reaching up high or low on shelves using a reacher tool to get objects without straining.

Safety and accident prevention at home depend on routinely evaluating the surroundings for possible risks and making the required corrections. Seeking advice from occupational therapists or home safety specialists can be quite beneficial when it comes to making efficient house changes that are customized for each person.

Keeping Yourself Independent Despite Osteoporosis

For those who have osteoporosis, maintaining their independence is crucial, even with the physical obstacles and limits that the condition may bring.

It is still possible to enjoy an independent and fulfilled life with the right techniques and help.

Staying independent requires taking a proactive approach to managing osteoporosis.

To maintain bone density and muscle strength, this entails following recommended treatment regimens, eating a balanced diet high in calcium and vitamin D, and exercising frequently.

By making up for physical constraints, the use of adapted equipment and assistive gadgets can also encourage independence. Wheelchairs, walkers, and canes are examples of devices that can improve mobility and make it easier and safer for people to carry out daily duties.

Furthermore, sustaining social links and participating in worthwhile pursuits are essential components of retaining autonomy and general well-being.

Engaging in pastimes, volunteering, or joining support groups can offer a feeling of direction and camaraderie, diminishing emotions of seclusion or reliance.

Maintaining good communication with medical providers is essential for controlling osteoporosis and resolving any issues or problems that may come up.

Appropriate evaluations and candid discussions with physicians, PTs, and other healthcare team members may guarantee that treatment regimens are tailored to each patient's needs.

Keeping one's independence in the face of osteoporosis requires developing a positive outlook and resilience. Putting an emphasis on one's skills, making reasonable goals, and acknowledging all successes—no matter how minor—can inspire people to overcome challenges and fully embrace life.

Asking For Help From Family And Friends And Medical Experts

It takes the assistance of loved ones and medical professionals to manage the complications of osteoporosis. Developing a robust support system can be of great help in controlling the illness and enhancing quality of life.

Obtaining advice from medical specialists such as physicians, nurses, and physical therapists is crucial in creating a successful treatment plan according to individual requirements.

These experts may provide knowledge, direction, and tailored advice on how to treat osteoporosis, including diet plans, exercise regimens, and lifestyle adjustments.

To cope with osteoporosis, it can be quite helpful to ask loved ones for support and understanding in addition to professional help.

In addition to providing emotional support and useful assistance with everyday tasks, family members, friends, and carers can go with patients to therapy or medical visits.

In order to make sure that each person's requirements are recognized and met, open communication is essential with loved ones as well as healthcare providers.

In order to manage osteoporosis, connections can be strengthened and a sense of teamwork can be promoted by sharing concerns, asking for assistance when necessary, and expressing gratitude for the support received.

Joining online networks or support groups for people with osteoporosis can also foster a sense of community and solidarity.

Making connections with people who have gone through similar things as you can provide support, encouragement, and insightful advice on how to deal with the difficulties of the illness.

In general, getting help from loved ones and medical professionals is crucial for controlling osteoporosis and preserving general health.

Through the establishment of a robust support system and proactive self-care practices, individuals can effectively manage their osteoporosis journey with increased resilience and confidence.

CHAPTER SIX

OSTEOPOROSIS AND EXERCISE

Exercises That Are Good for Bone Health

Not all workouts are made equal when it comes to bone health. Certain exercise regimens are especially helpful in building stronger bones and lowering the risk of osteoporosis.

Weight-bearing activities are great because they force the body to fight against gravity, which promotes bone density and growth. Examples of these workouts include walking, running, dancing, and trekking. The tension from these actions causes the bones to change, gradually growing stronger.

Exercises including strength training are also crucial for preserving bone health. Strengthening bones is supported by muscle mass, which can be developed and maintained by weightlifting and resistance band use. To maximize your bone health, concentrate on workouts like squats, lunges, and push-ups that engage main muscle groups.

routines for balance and coordination are just as important for preventing fractures and falls as weight-bearing and strength-training routines, particularly for older persons. Exercises like tai chi, yoga, and Pilates are great for enhancing posture, balance, and stability—all of which lower the risk of fractures and falls.

Finally, remember to perform flexibility exercises. In order to preserve general mobility and lower the risk of injury, stretching exercises can assist increase joint mobility and range of motion. To maintain the flexibility and health of your muscles and joints, include stretching exercises in your daily routine.

Establishing A Secure Workout Schedule

Safety needs to be the first consideration when designing an activity program for osteoporosis.

It's critical to select exercises that are suitable for your current level of fitness and health and to progressively increase the duration and intensity of your workouts over time.

Walking and swimming are good low-impact workouts to start with. As your strength and endurance increase, progressively move on to more difficult routines.

Before beginning any new exercise program, especially if you have osteoporosis or other medical issues, speak with your healthcare provider or a certified fitness professional. They can assist you in developing a customized workout program that takes into consideration your unique requirements and constraints.

Exercise with osteoporosis requires paying attention to your body and avoiding painful or uncomfortable activities. When exercising, stop right away if you suffer any strange symptoms, such as dizziness, shortness of breath, or chest pain, and get medical help if needed.

you lower the chance of injury, make sure you focus on correct form and technique in addition to selecting the appropriate workout programs. Consider consulting a licensed physical therapist or personal trainer for advice and training if you're not sure how to carry out a specific exercise correctly.

Finally, to assist avoid injuries and lessen muscular pain, remember to warm up before exercising and cool down afterward. Light aerobic activity for a few minutes, followed by some mild stretching, can assist your body get ready for exercise and aid in recuperation afterward.

Exercise Guidelines For People With Osteoporosis

Even while exercise is typically good for bone health, those with osteoporosis should take extra care to lower their chance of damage. Steer clear of high-impact exercises that require abrupt movements or jumping as these might raise the risk of fractures, particularly in people with brittle bones.

Instead, concentrate on low-impact activities like cycling, walking, swimming, or utilizing an elliptical machine that is easier on the bones and joints. These are safer options for those with osteoporosis since they offer the advantages of exercise without placing undue strain on the bones.

Exercises that require twisting or bending forward at the waist should be avoided if you have osteoporosis because they raise the risk of compression fractures in the spine. Rather, choose activities like Pilates or yoga that enhance spinal stability and alignment. These can help with posture and lower the chance of vertebral fractures.

Avoiding lifting large weights is another precaution to remember, particularly if you have fractures related to osteoporosis or bone loss in your spine. To develop strength without too stressing your bones, opt for smaller weights and concentrate on completing more repetitions.

Lastly, exercise with caution on uneven or slick surfaces as these might heighten the risk of fractures and falls, particularly for those who already have osteoporosis. If you want more stability and support throughout your workouts, think about utilizing walking aids or handrails as helpful equipment. Choose a level, sturdy terrain.

Combining Strength And Balance Training

An osteoporosis exercise program must include both balance and strength training since it lowers the risk of fractures and falls by enhancing muscle strength, stability, and posture. You can lower your risk of falling and enhance proprioception—the body's knowledge of its position in space—by including balancing exercises in your routine.

Over time, exercises like heel-to-toe walking, standing on one leg, and balancing on uneven surfaces (like a foam pad or balance board) can help test your balance and increase stability. For best results, try to incorporate balancing exercises into your program two or three times a week.

Strength training is equally important for those who have osteoporosis since it promotes bone health and lowers the risk of fractures by helping to maintain and grow muscle mass.

Concentrate on activities that work the main muscular groups, such as push-ups, squats, and lunges. You can intensify these exercises by using resistance bands or your body weight.

It's crucial to begin strength training with small weights while dealing with osteoporosis and to progressively increase the resistance as your strength increases.

To prevent injury, make sure you employ the right form and technique, and pay attention to your body to prevent overdoing it.

Incorporating balance and strength training activities into your regimen will assist improve general physical function and quality of life, minimizing the risk of falls and fractures linked with osteoporosis.

For optimal results, maintain a regular training schedule and progressively increase the level of intensity and difficulty of your activities over time.

Exercises for Flexibility to Preserve Mobility

Exercises for flexibility are a crucial part of any osteoporosis fitness program because they increase the range of motion, flexibility, and joint mobility while lowering the risk of injury and enhancing physical function. Stretching exercises will help you maintain or increase your flexibility, which will make it simpler to go about your everyday business and lower your chance of fractures and falls.

Make an effort to stretch the main muscular groups in your body, such as your hamstrings, quadriceps, calves, chest, shoulders, and back. Breathe deeply and hold each stretch for 15 to 30 seconds, extending gently to the point of tension but not pain.

Try to incorporate flexibility exercises into your regimen at least twice a week by repeating each stretch 2-4 times on each side.

Consider using dynamic stretching exercises like arm circles, torso twists, and leg swings in your program in addition to static stretching.

By preparing your muscles and joints for physical activity and enhancing joint mobility, dynamic stretching lowers your chance of injury.

To enhance blood flow and improve flexibility, warm up your muscles before completing any flexibility exercises with brisk cardio workouts like walking or cycling.

Warming up correctly before beginning a stretching program is important because extending cold muscles can raise the risk of injury.

Including flexibility exercises in your routine can help increase overall physical function, decrease stiffness, and improve mobility. T

his will make it simpler to go about your everyday activities and lower your risk of osteoporosis-related falls and fractures. To prevent overstretching and injury, stick to a stretching regimen and pay attention to your body.

CHAPTER SEVEN

SUMMARY AND EXPOSURE TO CANCER

Foods And Supplements High In Calcium

A sufficient intake of calcium is essential for maintaining bone health and preventing osteoporosis. Thankfully, there are many delectable and abundant foods high in calcium. In addition to the well-known dairy products—milk, yogurt, and cheese—you should also consider non-dairy alternatives such as almonds, tofu, leafy greens (kale, collard greens), and fortified drinks or cereals. You can increase your calcium intake by a large amount by including these foods in your daily diet.

Additionally helpful are supplements, particularly for those who might find it difficult to obtain adequate calcium from diet alone. There are several types of calcium supplements available, such as calcium citrate and carbonate. It's critical to adhere to the dosage recommendations made by your healthcare professional because excessive calcium consumption might cause negative effects and impede the absorption of other nutrients.

Sources And Dosages Of Vitamin D

In order to support bone health, vitamin D and calcium function together. It helps keep blood levels of calcium and phosphate at appropriate levels and facilitates the absorption of calcium from the intestines. Although vitamin D is naturally found in sunlight, many individuals don't get enough of it because of things like living in northern latitudes, spending more time indoors, or frequently wearing sunscreen.

Egg yolks, fortified dairy products, fortified cereals, fatty fish (salmon, mackerel), and sunshine exposure are dietary sources of vitamin D. Supplementation may be required for people who find it difficult to get enough vitamin D from food and sunshine. Supplements with different levels of vitamin D are generally accessible. Based on your particular circumstances, your healthcare practitioner can advise you on the right dosage.

Protein's Importance For Healthy Bones

Although protein is frequently linked to the health of muscles, it is also essential for strong and healthy bones. The protein collagen, which is present in bone tissue, gives things shape and support. Furthermore, bone remodeling—the ongoing disintegration and reconstruction of bone tissue—requires protein.

Bone health can be supported by including high-quality protein sources in your diet, such as fish, poultry, beans, almonds, seeds, and lean meats. Spread your protein consumption throughout the day through meals and snacks to get a balanced intake. A sufficient protein diet is essential for maintaining muscle mass and lowering the incidence of fractures, especially for older persons.

Foods To Restrict Or Stay Away From

While some foods can strengthen bones and promote bone health, others may have the reverse impact and weaken or cause bone loss. Foods high in sodium, for instance, may cause an increase in the excretion of calcium in the urine, which over time may cause a deficiency of calcium in the bones. Fast food meals, processed foods, canned soups, and salty snacks are frequently found to contain high amounts of sodium.

In a similar vein, drinking too much alcohol can harm your bones. Alcohol can alter hormone levels that are important in bone remodeling and interfere with the body's ability to absorb calcium. Reducing alcohol consumption to moderate amounts (one drink for women and up to two for men) will help lessen these effects and improve bone health in general.

Organising Meals For Maximum Bone Strength

Making a food plan that puts an emphasis on nutrients that build bones doesn't have to be difficult. Start by including a range of foods high in calcium, protein, and vitamin D in your meals and snacks. Leafy greens, dairy or plant-based calcium sources, lean meats, legumes, nuts, and seeds, as well as fatty fish, should all be included.

To make sure you're getting a wide range of nutrients, when you plan your meals, strive for balance and variety. Incorporate an abundance of fruits and vegetables to obtain antioxidants and micronutrients that promote general well-being. Remember to stay hydrated as well; consuming enough water is crucial to keeping strong bones and general health.

You can maintain the health of your bones and lower your risk of osteoporosis and fractures by being proactive with your diet and meal planning. Seek advice from a qualified dietician or other healthcare professional for individualized recommendations based on your unique requirements and preferences.

CHAPTER EIGHT

OVERCOMING OSTEOPOROSIS AT DIFFERENT PHASES OF LIFE

Osteoporosis In Adolescents And Children

Recognising Osteoporosis Early: Although less frequent in younger adults than in older adults, osteoporosis in children and adolescents can have serious long-term effects on bone health. Bone mass grows significantly during these formative years, peaking in early adulthood. Nevertheless, a few things may obstruct this process, decreasing bone density and raising the risk of fractures.

Causes and Risk Factors: A number of variables influence the development of osteoporosis in kids and teenagers. Genetic predisposition, hormonal imbalances, dietary deficiencies (particularly in calcium and vitamin D), chronic illnesses, specific drugs, and lifestyle choices like excessive alcohol and tobacco use or physical inactivity are a few examples of these.

Evaluation and Diagnosis: Healthcare providers must carefully assess patients in order to diagnose osteoporosis in children and adolescents.

In order to do this, a physical examination, an evaluation of medical history, and specialized bone density tests like dual-energy X-ray absorptiometry (DEXA) is usually performed. Blood tests may also be performed in order to rule out underlying medical diseases that could be causing problems with bone health.

Treatment and Management: The goal of managing osteoporosis in children and teenagers is to reduce the risk of fracture and maximize bone health. Treatment plans frequently combine dietary changes, lifestyle adjustments, encouraging physical exercise, and, in certain situations, pharmaceuticals. During this key phase, it is imperative to provide sufficient intake of calcium and vitamin D through diet and supplements to maintain bone development.

Encouraging physical exercise is crucial for promoting bone health as it helps to form and maintain strong bones. Weight-bearing activities like dancing, jogging, and walking support the development of new bone and increase bone density. In addition, boosting outdoor activities, restricting screen time, and abstaining from sedentary behaviors can all improve general bone health.

Educational and Supportive Measures: It is critical to teach kids, teens, and their families the value of bone health. Giving advice on diet, exercise, and lifestyle choices can enable people to actively manage their risk of osteoporosis. Additionally, providing tools and assistance to manage the psychological and emotional effects of having a chronic illness can improve well-being in general.

Young Adults And Middle-Aged People's Osteoporosis

Managing Bone Health During the Early Adult Years:

A crucial time for preserving ideal bone health and avoiding osteoporosis in later life is young adulthood and middle age. People usually reach their optimum bone mass during these phases, which establishes the groundwork for skeletal strength in later life. On the other hand, environmental variables and lifestyle decisions might affect fracture risk and bone density.

Modifiable Risk Factors: A number of modifiable risk factors can affect a person's bone health in middle age and early adulthood. These include a sedentary lifestyle, smoking, excessive alcohol use, poor calcium and vitamin D intake, inadequate nutrition, and some medical diseases or drugs that interfere with bone metabolism. Early intervention to address these factors can reduce the incidence of osteoporosis.

Early detection and prevention: Although young adults and middle-aged people may not think much about osteoporosis, taking preventative measures can greatly lower the chance of developing the condition later in life.

Frequent health screenings can detect early indicators of bone loss and enable timely management, including bone density tests for high-risk patients. Moreover, maintaining bone density and strength requires embracing healthy lifestyle practices like quitting smoking, eating a balanced diet, and getting regular exercise.

Career and Lifestyle Considerations: During young adulthood and middle age, bone health can be impacted by occupational and lifestyle choices. Over time, the risk of fracture may increase for some occupations or activities that involve physical strain or repetitive stress. As a result, when participating in such activities, people should take safety measures to preserve their bones, such as using appropriate ergonomics, wearing safety gear, and taking regular rests to avoid overuse injuries.

Health Promotion Strategies: Diverse strategies are needed to promote bone health in young adults and middle-aged people. Companies, medical professionals, and neighborhood associations can work together to increase public knowledge of osteoporosis risk factors and protective strategies. Providing resources for healthy living, educational workshops, and workplace wellness programs can encourage people to put their bone health first.

Long-Term Planning and Continuity of Care: Although osteoporosis may seem unafraid in middle age and young adulthood, establishing the framework for preventative care paves the way for aging in a healthy manner. Continuity of care can be guaranteed by incorporating bone-friendly practices into everyday activities and being cautious about routine health check-ups. People can protect their bone health and have more energy as they age by being proactive in their early years.

Osteoporosis During Breastfeeding And Pregnancy

Maternal Bone Health Considerations: The health of a mother's bones is particularly challenged during pregnancy and nursing. Women experience major physiological changes throughout these stages, including higher calcium requirements to support nursing and fetal growth.

The body of the mother adjusts to meet these needs, but if sufficient nutritional assistance is not received, bone loss may occur.

Calcium Requirements and Supplementation: To support the bone health of both the mother and the fetus, it is essential to maintain an appropriate calcium intake during pregnancy and lactation.

Women who are expecting or nursing should try to get enough calcium from their diets by eating dairy products, leafy greens, fortified foods, and supplements if needed. Healthcare professionals may suggest calcium supplements in light of a patient's unique requirements and risk factors.

Exercise and Weight-Bearing Activities: Maintaining bone density and strength throughout pregnancy and lactation can be facilitated by regular physical activity, which includes weight-bearing activities.

To guarantee safety and appropriateness, pregnant and nursing women should speak with their healthcare providers prior to beginning or altering an exercise program.

Walking, swimming, and prenatal yoga are examples of low-impact exercises that can be quite beneficial without putting too much strain on the joints.

Nutritional Support and Counselling: During pregnancy and lactation, nutritional counseling is essential for maximizing the health of the mother's bones.

To improve bone density and general well-being, healthcare providers can provide advice on food choices, supplements, and lifestyle alterations. For calcium absorption and bone metabolism, adequate vitamin D consumption is also necessary, especially for women who have restricted sun exposure or dietary limitations.

Postpartum Bone Recovery: Hormonal shifts and physiological adaptations following childbirth might cause women to temporarily lose bone density. As dietary requirements return to normal and hormone levels stabilize, postpartum bone healing usually happens gradually. To avoid difficulties, women who have high-risk characteristics or pre-existing osteoporosis may need greater monitoring and assistance.

Finding a Careful Balance between the Needs of the Baby and the Mother: Managing the health of the mother's bones during pregnancy and lactation entails finding a careful balance between the mother's needs and those of the child. Healthcare professionals can provide advice on how to maximize calcium intake without sacrificing the health of mothers or the objectives of breastfeeding. Promoting the health and vibrancy of mother and child requires continual support and collaborative decision-making.

Osteoporosis In Seniors And Older Adults

Age-Related Bone Changes: As people age, their bone density and structure alter, which raises their risk of fractures and osteoporosis. Due to age-related decreases in calcium absorption and bone turnover, as well as hormonal changes and decreased physical activity, older individuals and seniors are more susceptible to bone loss. Comprehending these aging-related alterations is essential for efficient osteoporosis treatment.

Strategies for Fracture Prevention: One of the main objectives of treating osteoporosis in the elderly is preventing fractures.

This entails all-encompassing tactics designed to lower the risk of falls, strengthen bones, and treat underlying medical issues that fuel bone fragility.

Modifications to the surroundings, exercises for strength and balance, medication administration, and routine evaluations of hearing and vision are a few examples of possible interventions.

Medication Management and Adherence: For older individuals and seniors treating osteoporosis, pharmacological therapies are essential. To lower the risk of fracture and increase bone density, doctors may recommend drugs such as hormone treatment, bisphosphonates, or selective estrogen receptor modulators (SERMs). But especially for this group, making sure that medication is taken as prescribed and keeping an eye out for any negative effects are crucial factors to take into account.

Nutrition and a Bone-Friendly Diet: Sustaining general well-being and bone health in elders and older adults requires adequate nutrition. Foods high in calcium, vitamin D supplements, and protein sources are especially crucial for maintaining muscle mass and bone density.

A balanced diet that emphasizes whole grains, fruits, vegetables, and healthy fats can also supply vital nutrients and support the best possible bone health.

Fall Prevention and Safety Measures: Seniors with osteoporosis who want to lower their risk of fracture must take immediate action to prevent falls.

Fall risk and related injuries can be reduced by putting fall prevention measures into practice, such as clearing out potential dangers from the home, adding grab bars and handrails, utilizing assistive technology, and engaging in mobility and balancing exercises.

Multidisciplinary Care Strategy: Treating osteoporosis in the elderly and other senior citizens frequently calls for a multidisciplinary strategy including medical specialists from different fields.

Together, geriatricians, orthopedists, physical therapists, dietitians, and pharmacists evaluate patients' needs, create individualized treatment programs, and oversee follow-up care.

This all-encompassing strategy fosters independence and a high quality of life while addressing the many health problems related to aging.

CHAPTER NINE

COMMON QUESTIONS AND ANSWERS

Is It Possible To Regain Bone Mass?

With its weakening of the bones, osteoporosis begs the urgent question: Is it reversible? Even though a natural aspect of aging is the loss of bone density, this process can be slowed down or even stopped.

On the other hand, osteoporosis reversal is more difficult. The main goals of effective management strategies are to lower the risk of fractures and stop additional loss of bone density.

Fundamental lifestyle changes include frequent exercise, particularly weight-bearing and resistance training, and a well-balanced diet high in calcium and vitamin D. Furthermore, drugs recommended by medical professionals can strengthen bones and reduce the chance of fractures. But in extreme cases, it might not be possible to completely reverse osteoporosis, which highlights the significance of early detection and proactive care.

Do Any All-Natural Treatments For Osteoporosis?

In addition to traditional osteoporosis therapies, natural remedies can improve general bone health and lower the risk of fractures. To keep bone density, one must consume enough calcium and vitamin D through food or supplements. Dairy products, leafy greens, almonds, and fortified foods are among the foods high in calcium. Vitamin D can be obtained mostly from sunshine exposure, while supplements are also an option if needed. Frequent exercise, especially weight-bearing and muscle-strengthening activities, helps to increase bone density and lower the chance of falling. Further research is required to confirm the efficiency and safety of certain herbal supplements, such as red clover, black cohosh, and soy isoflavones, for the treatment of osteoporosis, as they may have potential bone-protective benefits.

How Do Guys Get Osteoporosis?

Though more commonly linked to women, osteoporosis can also afflict men, but less frequently. Because men's bones are usually denser and thicker than women's, osteoporosis may not develop as quickly in men.

But as men become older, their bone density progressively decreases, raising their risk of osteoporosis and fractures. Men can develop osteoporosis due to a variety of factors, including insufficient testosterone, long-term health issues, certain drugs, smoking, heavy alcohol use, and a sedentary lifestyle. For men, osteoporosis-related fractures can have major repercussions, including diminished quality of life, increased mortality, and disability.

Therefore, the key to lessening the impact of this condition is increasing awareness of osteoporosis in males, promoting preventative measures, and enabling early detection through bone density testing.

Can Osteoporosis Be Inherited?

A person's genetic makeup greatly influences their likelihood of acquiring osteoporosis. Although having a family history of osteoporosis does not ensure one will get the disease, it can make one more susceptible. Osteoporosis risk is influenced by a number of hereditary variables that affect bone turnover, density, and structure.

Gene variations that impact bone health and predispose people to osteoporosis include those linked to vitamin D receptors, collagen synthesis, bone metabolism, and estrogen receptors.

But environmental factors including nutrition, exercise, smoking, alcohol use, and medication also play important roles in the development of osteoporosis; hereditary predisposition is only one piece of the picture. Knowing how genetics and lifestyle variables interact can help people identify their risk and take preventative measures against osteoporosis.

What Recent Developments Exist In The Field Of Osteoporosis Research?

Research on osteoporosis is a dynamic topic that is always developing thanks to new findings and developments. Innovative treatment methods, diagnostic tools, and preventive measures are the main focus of recent advancements in the fight against the increasing global osteoporosis burden. The creation of new drugs that specifically target bone metabolic pathways in an effort to increase bone density and lower the risk of fracture is one exciting field of research. Furthermore, a more precise evaluation of bone quality and fracture risk is now possible thanks to developments in imaging technology, such as trabecular bone score (TBS) and high-resolution peripheral quantitative computed tomography (HR-pQCT). In order to forecast osteoporosis risk and personalize treatment regimens, researchers are also investigating the roles that biomarkers, epigenetics, and genetics may play. Personalized medicine and precision approaches to osteoporosis therapy are also being paved by the innovative work being done in the field of osteoporosis research thanks to interdisciplinary cooperation between scientists, clinicians, and industry partners.

www.ingramcontent.com/pod-product-compliance
Lightning Source LLC
Chambersburg PA
CBHW071837210526
45479CB00001B/183